Basic Notes in Psychopharmacol

The views expressed in this book reflect the experience of the author and are not necessarily those of Lundbeck Ltd. Any products referred to by the author should only be used as recommended in the manufacturers' data sheets.

Previous books by the same author

Levi, M. I. (1987). MCQs for the MRCPsych Part I. (Lancaster: MTP Press)

Levi, M. I. (1988). MCQs for the MRCPsych Part II. (Lancaster: Kluwer Academic Publishers)

Levi, M. I. (1988). SAQs for the MRCPsych Part II. (Lancaster: Kluwer Academic Publishers)

Levi, M. I. (1992). PMPs for the MRCPsych Part II. (Lancaster: Kluwer Academic Publishers)

Levi, M. I. (1996). Basic Notes in Psychotherapy. (Newbury: Petroc Press)

Levi, M. I. (1997). MCQs for the MRCPsych (Newbury: Petroc Press)

Levi, M. I. (2003). Basic Notes in Psychiatry, Third Edition (Newbury: Petroc Press)

Basic Notes in Psychopharmacology

by

Dr Michael I. Levi MB BS MRCPsych
Consultant Psychiatrist
Bradford District Care Trust
Horton Park Centre
Bradford, West Yorkshire, UK

THIRD EDITION

Radcliffe Publishing
Oxford • San Francisco

Radcliffe Publishing Ltd
18 Marcham Road
Abingdon
Oxon OX14 1AA
United Kingdom

www.radcliffe-oxford.com
Electronic catalogue and worldwide online ordering facility.

First Edition 1993 (published by Kluwer Academic Publishers)
Second Edition 1998 (published by Petroc Press)

British Library Cataloguing in Publication Data

A catalogue record for this book is available from the British Library.

ISBN 1 85775 671 1

Typeset by Richard Powell Editorial and Production Services, Basingstoke, Hants

Printed and bound in the United Kingdom by Cromwell Press

Contents

Foreword to the Third Edition

Now in its third edition, this handy book has lost none of its straightforward approach and provides a concise, easy to understand, quick reference source to what can be a potentially confusing area. Updated to reflect current practice and to include the new drugs that have been launched since the last edition, it continues to be a valuable guide to prescribers.

Alistair Tinto, MCMHP
(Member of College of Mental Health Pharmacists)
Lead Pharmacist Community and Mental Health
Bradford Hospitals NHS Trust

Preface to the Third Edition

Following the popularity of the second edition, I was encouraged to write this new edition for junior hospital psychiatrists, general practitioners and medical students.

I have completely updated the book to include new psychotropic drugs that have been launched in the UK since the appearance of the second edition in 1998. I have also reviewed all the drugs covered in the second edition and updated these entries, where appropriate, in the light of current knowledge.

2004 M.I.L.

Introduction

The purpose of writing this book is to provide a concise summary of psychopharmacology in the form of notes. The drugs discussed in this book are those considered by the author to be the most important drugs that the practising physician needs to know about. The aim is to provide the principal mode of action, indications and adverse effects of the drugs covered. I have based these notes on what is generally regarded to be the most comprehensive textbook[1] for the MRCPsych examination. These notes represent my own view of current clinical practice.

The book is intended to have wide readership – particularly among junior hospital psychiatrists, general practitioners and medical students. In addition, the book will also be useful to psychiatric nurses, psychiatric social workers, psychiatric occupational therapists and clinical psychologists.

Reference

1. Gelder M, Lopez-Ibor JJ, Andreasen N, eds. New Oxford Textbook of Psychiatry. 2003: Oxford University Press.

CHAPTER 1

Hypnotic and Anxiolytic Drugs

I. BENZODIAZEPINES

(a) Mode of action

1. GABA (γ-aminobutyric acid) agonists; act at benzodiazepine BZ_1- and BZ_2-receptors which are located postsynaptically throughout the brain at GABA-ergic synapses.
2. There are three subtypes of benzodiazepine receptors:
   (i) Omega-1 – mediates hypnotic effect of drug
   (ii) Omega-2 – mediates anxiolytic effect of drug
   (iii) Omega-3 – mediates myorelaxant effect of drug.
   Benzodiazepines act on all three receptor subtypes and therefore have muscle relaxant, anxiolytic and hypnotic effects.

(b) Indications

1. Transient insomnia in those who normally sleep well – if a benzodiazepine is indicated, use one that has a short half-life with little or no hangover effect and only prescribe 1 or 2 doses of the drug, e.g. lormetazepam; dose range 0.5 mg nocte to 1.5 mg nocte.
2. Anxiety disorders (generalised anxiety disorder and panic disorder) – provide symptomatic relief of severe anxiety in the short term (should not be prescribed for more than 2–4 weeks), e.g. diazepam; dose range 2 mg t.d.s. increased if necessary to 15–30 mg daily in divided doses. The use of an antidepressant drug should also be considered in this situation (see later).

3. Phobic anxiety disorders – provide some immediate relief of phobic symptoms in the short term.
4. Obsessive compulsive disorders – provide some short-term symptomatic relief (should not be prescribed for more than 2–4 weeks' duration).
5. Acute organic disorder:
   (i) May be used during the night-time to help the patient sleep.
   (ii) In the special case of hepatic failure – may be used during the day-time to calm the patient despite their sedative effects, since they are less likely to precipitate coma – cf. haloperidol (which is the usual drug of choice to calm such patients).
   (iii) In the special case of alcohol withdrawal – chlordiazepoxide is the most suitable drug.
6. Chronic organic disorder – may be used to alleviate anxiety.
7. Barbiturate dependence – used to cover the withdrawal symptoms from barbiturates.
8. Acutely disturbed behaviour – if an antipsychotic drug alone fails to bring the situation under control, they may be given in addition a slow intramuscular injection of 2 mg of lorazepam, if necessary repeated 2 hours later.
9. Akathisia.

(c) Adverse effects

1. Both psychic and physical dependence occur.
2. Chronic benzodiazepine dependence – often manifests features of benzodiazepine intoxication, which are:
   (i) Unsteadiness of gait.
   (ii) Dysarthria.

   (iii) Drowsiness.
   (iv) Nystagmus.
3. Withdrawal effects from benzodiazepines:
   (i) Rebound insomnia.
   (ii) Tremor.
   (iii) Anxiety.
   (iv) Restlessness.
   (v) Appetite disturbance.
   (vi) Weight loss.
   (vii) Sweating.
   (viii) Convulsions.
   (ix) Confusion.
   (x) Toxic psychosis.
   (xi) A condition resembling delirium tremens.

4. Benzodiazepines – cf. barbiturates. Advantages of benzodiazepines:
   (i) Milder side-effects – including less risk of respiratory depression.
   (ii) Less severe physical dependence.
   (iii) Less dangerous in overdosage.
   (iv) Less likely to interact with other drugs – as induction of hepatic microsomal enzymes does not occur to the same extent.

II. BARBITURATES

(a) Mode of action

GABA potentiators; do not act at benzodiazepine receptors; may have specific binding sites elsewhere on the neuronal membrane.

(b) Indications

1. Severe intractable insomnia in patients already taking barbiturates – even in such patients, an attempt to slowly withdraw the barbiturate should be considered, covering the withdrawal syndrome with a benzodiazepine.
2. Dissociative (conversion) disorders – classically, abreaction was brought about by an intravenous injection of small amounts of amylobarbitone sodium. In the resulting state, the patient is encouraged to relive the stressful events that provoked the hysteria, and to express the accompanying emotions. Now, such abreaction can be initiated more safely by a slow intravenous injection of 10 mg of diazepam.

(c) Adverse effects

1. Both psychic and physical dependence occur.
2. Chronic barbiturate dependence – often manifests features of barbiturate intoxication, which are:
   (i) Slurred speech.
   (ii) Incoherence.
   (iii) Dullness.
   (iv) Drowsiness.
   (v) Nystagmus.
   (vi) Depression.
3. Withdrawal effects from barbiturates:
   (i) Clouding of consciousness.
   (ii) Disorientation.
   (iii) Hallucinations.
   (iv) Major seizures.
   (v) Anxiety.
   (vi) Restlessness.
   (vii) Pyrexia.

(viii) Tremulousness.
(ix) Insomnia.
(x) Hypotension.
(xi) Nausea.
(xii) Vomiting.
(xiii) Anorexia.
(xiv) Twitching.
(xv) A condition resembling delirium tremens.

4. Drug interactions – induction of hepatic microsomal enzymes leads to increased metabolism of:
   (i) The oral contraceptive pill.
   (ii) Corticosteroids.
   (iii) Warfarin.
   (iv) Tricyclic antidepressants.
   (v) Most antipsychotic drugs.
   (vi) Cyclosporin.
   (vii) Theophylline.

III. CHLORAL DERIVATIVES

(a) Mode of action

GABA potentiators.

(b) Indications

Short-term treatment of insomnia e.g. chloral betaine; rarely used now.

(c) Adverse effects

Abuse potential – therefore should not be prescribed for more than 1–2 weeks' duration.

IV. OTHERS

1. CHLORMETHIAZOLE

(a) Mode of action

GABA potentiator.

(b) Indications

In the management of alcohol withdrawal for inpatients only, chlormethiazole may be prescribed in either of two ways:

1. On an as-required basis, i.e. flexibly according to the patient's symptoms.
2. On a reducing regimen basis, i.e. on a fixed 6-hourly regimen of gradually decreasing dosage over 6–9 days.

N.B.: *Alternatively, chlordiazepoxide may be used in the management of alcohol withdrawal – this has the advantage over chlormethiazole of being less addictive and being less dangerous if taken in combination with alcohol.*

(c) Adverse effect

May cause acute cardiac arrest or acute respiratory arrest if taken in combination with alcohol.

2. β-BLOCKERS

(a) Mode of action

Block β-adrenoreceptors in the heart, peripheral vasculature, bronchi, liver and pancreas and brain (although CNS penetration is poor).

(b) Indications

Limited use in treating anxiety disorders in which palpitations, sweating or tremor are the most troublesome symptoms, i.e. those anxiety disorders with predominantly somatic symptoms, e.g. propranolol; dose range 40 mg b.d. (or 80 mg SR) to 40 mg t.d.s.
N.B.: *β-Blockers have little effect on subjective feelings of anxiety.*

(c) Adverse effects

Contraindicated in patients with:

1. Asthma.
2. A history of obstructive airways disease.
3. Uncontrolled heart failure.
4. Second- or third-degree heart block.

3. BUSPIRONE

(a) Mode of action

1. Thought to act at specific serotonin (5HT1A) presynaptic autoreceptors – as a partial agonist.
2. Response to treatment may take up to 2 weeks – similar to antidepressant drugs.

(b) Indications

1. Short-term treatment (up to several months) of generalised anxiety disorder; usual dose range 5 mg t.d.s. to 10 mg t.d.s.; maximum dose of 15 mg t.d.s.; long term efficacy is untested.
2. May be useful in the treatment of resistant depression – as an augmenting agent to SSRIs (by enhancing serotonin accumulation within the synapse).
3. May be useful in the treatment of obsessive compulsive

disorder – as an augmenting agent to SSRIs.

(c) Adverse effects

1. Physical dependence and abuse liability low.
2. Non-toxic augmenting agent, cf. lithium carbonate.
3. Does not potentiate the effects of alcohol, cf. benzodiazepines, which do.
4. Lacks sedative and myorelaxant properties of benzodiazepines.

4. ZOPICLONE

(a) Mode of action

1. The first cyclopyrrolone.
2. GABA potentiator – although not a benzodiazepine, it acts on benzodiazepine receptors which are located postsynaptically throughout the brain at GABA-ergic synapses.
3. Acts on Omega-1 and Omega-2 receptor subtypes and therefore has anxiolytic and hypnotic effects.

(b) Indications

1. Transient insomnia in those who normally sleep well – as an alternative to a benzodiazepine; dosage 7.5 mg nocte in adults.
2. For short-term use only (preferably only 1 or 2 doses).

(c) Adverse effects

Since it acts on benzodiazepine receptors, it may give rise to the problems of physical dependence as observed in benzodiazepines if used for long-term treatment.

5. ZOLPIDEM

(a) Mode of action

1. The first imidazopyridine.
2. GABA potentiator – although not a benzodiazepine, it acts on benzodiazepine receptors which are located postsynaptically throughout the brain at GABA-ergic synapses.
3. Acts on Omega-1 receptor subtype only and therefore has a pure hypnotic effect.

(b) Indications

1. Transient insomnia in those who normally sleep well – as an alternative to a benzodiazepine; dosage 10 mg nocte in adults.
2. For short-term use only (preferably only 1 or 2 doses).

(c) Adverse effect

1. Since it acts on one of the same receptor subtypes as benzodiazepines, it may give rise to the problems of physical dependence as observed in benzodiazepines if used for long-term treatment.
2. May have less abuse potential because it spares the Omega-2 receptor subtype, cf zopiclone.

---

6. ZALEPLON

(a) Mode of Action

Acts on the Omega-1 subtype of the central benzodiazepine's receptor – and therefore has a pure hypnotic effect.

(b) Indications

1. Insomnia (short term use).
2. Dosage 10 mg at bedtime or after going to bed if difficulty falling asleep; the latter is accounted for by the very short half life (duration of action) of Zaleplon.

(c) Adverse effect

May have less abuse potential because it spares the Omega-2 receptor subtype, cf. zopiclone.

CHAPTER 2

Antipsychotic Drugs

CLASSIFICATION

Conventional Antipsychotics
1. Chlorpromazine
2. Haloperidol
3. Trifluoperazine
4. Sulpiride
5. Pimozide
6. Zuclopenthixol Acetate

Atypical Antipsychotics
1. Risperidone
2. Olanzapine
3. Quetiapine
4. Amisulpride
5. Aripiprazole
6. Zotepine
7. Clozapine

Antipsychotic Depot Injections
1. Fluphenazine Decanoate
2. Flupenthixol Decanoate
3. Zuclopenthixol Decanoate
4. Haloperidol Decanoate
5. Pipothiazine Palmitate
6. IM Risperidone

CONVENTIONAL ANTIPSYCHOTICS

I. CHLORPROMAZINE

(a) Mode of action

1. Dopamine antagonist; blocks D_2-receptors in the meso-limbic cortical bundle – which mediates the anti-psychotic action of chlorpromazine.
2. It also has several other biochemical actions which mediate the side-effects of chlorpromazine:
   - (i) Dopamine blocking activity at other sites (see later).
   - (ii) Antiserotonergic activity.
   - (iii) α_1-Adrenergic receptor antagonist.
   - (iv) Muscarinic M_1-receptor antagonist.
   - (v) Histamine H_1-receptor antagonist.

(b) Indications

1. Schizophrenia:
   - (i) Control and maintenance therapy in schizophrenia (usual maintenance dose 50 mg b.d. to 100 mg t.d.s.; maximum dose 1 g daily in divided doses).
   - (ii) Chlorpromazine is more sedative and causes less extrapyramidal side-effects, cf. haloperidol – thus, chlorpromazine was the drug of choice for schizophrenia (before the advent of atypical antipsychotics).
2. Affective disorders:
   - (i) Control of the psychotic components of psychotic depression.
   - (ii) Usually brings the symptoms of acute mania under rapid control.

3. Persistent delusional disorder – symptoms are sometimes relieved.
4. Obsessive compulsive disorders – small doses of value when anxiolytic treatment is needed for more than the 2–4 weeks' duration for which benzodiazepines are prescribed.
5. Personality disorders – may be given for short periods at times of unusual stress.
6. Chronic organic disorder – alleviation of certain symptoms of dementia:
   (i) Anxiety.
   (ii) Overactivity.
   (iii) Delusions.
   (iv) Hallucinations.

N.B.: *Care is needed to find the optimal dose; in the elderly there are the special dangers of hypotension, atropinic effects and ECG changes – therefore haloperidol is preferred to chlorpromazine in the elderly.*

7. Behavioural disturbances – tranquillization and emergency control.
8. Severe anxiety – short-term adjunctive treatment.
9. Terminal disease.
10. Anti-emetic.
11. Intractable hiccup.

(c) Adverse effects

1. Extrapyramidal side-effects (EPSEs) – mediated by dopamine-blocking activity at D_2-receptors in the nigrostriatal pathway:
   (i) Acute dystonic reactions.
   (ii) Akathisia.
   (iii) Pseudoparkinsonism.
   (iv) Tardive dyskinesia.
2. Hyperprolactinaemia – mediated by dopamine blocking

activity at D_2 receptors in the tubero-infundibular system – galactorrhoea in both women and men.

3. Antiserotonergic side-effect: depression.
4. Antiadrenergic side-effects (due to blockade of α_1-adrenergic receptor):
   (i) Postural hypotension.
   (ii) Failure of ejaculation.
   (iii) Sedation.
5. Anticholinergic side-effects (due to blockade of muscarinic M_1-receptors):
   (i) Dry mouth.
   (ii) Blurred vision.
   (iii) Constipation.
   (iv) Urinary retention.
   (v) Tachycardia.
   (vi) Impotence.
   (vii) Exacerbation of glaucoma.
6. Antihistaminergic side-effect (due to blockade of histamine H_1-receptors): sedation.

N.B.: *Sedation is mainly mediated through anti-adrenergic activity.*

7. Impaired temperature regulation:
   (i) Hypothermia.
   (ii) Hyperpyrexia.
8. Neuroleptic malignant syndrome (NMS).
9. Bone marrow suppression – leucopenia.
10. Skin photosensitivity and pigmentation.
11. Cardiac arrhythmias.
12. Cholestatic jaundice.
13. Seizures (due to lowering of the convulsive threshold).
14. Weight gain.

II. HALOPERIDOL

(a) Mode of action

1. Greater dopamine blocking activity.
2. Less antiadrenergic activity.
3. Less anticholinergic activity.

(1–3: cf. chlorpromazine)

(b) Indications

1. Mania.
2. Treatment of acute organic disorder during the day-time.
3. Bringing acutely disturbed behaviour under immediate control – since it is less sedative and causes less postural hypotension than chlorpromazine.
4. Other non-affective psychoses.

(c) Adverse effects

1. More EPSE.
2. Less sedation.
3. Less postural hypotension.

(1–3: cf. chlorpromazine)

4. Less anticholinergic side-effects.
5. NMS.
6. Danger of severe EPSE with haloperidol if a daily dose in excess of 20 mg is combined with lithium carbonate at a serum level of greater than 0.8 mmol/l.
7. ECG changes at high dose – torsade de pointes.
8. Recently the maximum BNF recommended dose of haloperidol has been heavily reduced to:
   (i) 30 mg daily in divided doses if taken orally
   (ii) 18 mg daily in divided doses as an intramuscular injection.

   This is due to EPSE at higher doses.

III. TRIFLUOPERAZINE

(a) Mode of action

1. Greater dopamine blocking activity.
2. Less antiadrenergic activity.
3. Less anticholinergic activity.

} cf. chlorpromazine

(b) Indications

1. Useful in psychotic patients where sedation is undesirable (i.e. retarded psychotic patients) – since it is less sedative – cf. chlorpromazine.
2. Useful in psychotic patients with intractable auditory hallucinations; usual dose range 5 mg b.d. to 5 mg t.d.s.

(c) Adverse effects

1. More EPSE.
2. Less sedation.
3. Less postural hypotension.
4. Less anticholinergic side-effects.

} cf. chlorpromazine

IV. SULPIRIDE

(a) Mode of action

1. Low doses – thought to block presynaptic dopamine D_3- and D_4-autoreceptors.
2. High doses – blocks postsynaptic dopamine receptors; more specific blocker of D_2-receptors – cf. D_1-receptors.

(b) Indications

1. Low doses – may have an alerting effect on schizo-

phrenic patients with negative symptoms such as apathy and social withdrawal (optimum dosage 400 mg b.d.).

2. High doses – useful in schizophrenic patients with florid positive symptoms such as delusions and hallucinations (optimum dosage 800 mg b.d.).

(c) Adverse effects

1. Less EPSE – cf. chlorpromazine.
2. Less sedation – cf. chlorpromazine.
3. Tendency to cause galactorrhoea.

V. PIMOZIDE

(a) Mode of action

More specific blocker of D_3- and D_2-receptors – cf. chlorpromazine.

(b) Indication

Useful in monosymptomatic delusional psychosis – it is claimed that pimozide has success in specifically targeting monosymptomatic hypochondriacal delusions (dose range 4–16 mg daily).

N.B.: *Special caution is needed over rate of rise in daily doses.*

(c) Adverse effects

1. Less EPSE. } cf. chlorpromazine
2. Less sedation. }
3. Following reports of sudden unexplained death, CSM recommends:

(i) An ECG prior to commencing treatment in all patients.
(ii) ECGs at regular intervals in patients taking over 16 mg daily.
(iii) A review of the need for pimozide if arrhythmias develop.

VI. ZUCLOPENTHIXOL ACETATE

(a) Mode of action

Short-acting injection administered intramuscularly as an oily injection and rapidly released into the bloodstream.

(b) Indications

Useful for immediate management of acutely disturbed behaviour as an alternative to haloperidol since:

1. Zuclopenthixol acetate is more sedative than haloperidol.
2. These injections (maximum of four) are more easily administered to the patient, cf. trying to persuade such a patient to comply with regular oral or intramuscular haloperidol.

(c) Cautions

1. Treatment duration should not exceed 2 weeks with a maximum dosage of 150 mg for each injection per 24 hours, and a maximum dosage of 400 mg for each course of injections.
2. Must not be used on neuroleptic naïve patients, i.e. haloperidol should be tried first and been ineffective before considering zuclopenthixol acetate.

ATYPICAL ANTIPSYCHOTICS

RISPERIDONE

Introduced into the UK in 1993

(a) Mode of action

1. Potent dopamine D_2-receptor antagonist; in addition it has a regional preference for blocking D_2-receptors in the mesolimbic cortical bundle, cf. the nigrostriatal pathway.
2. Potent serotonin $5HT_{2A}$-receptor antagonist.
3. Low affinity for serotonin $5HT_{2C}$-receptors.
4. Potent α_1-adrenergic receptor antagonist.
5. No appreciable affinity for muscarinic M_1-receptors.
6. Low affinity for histamine H_1-receptors.

(b) Indications

1. Treatment of both the positive and negative symptoms of schizophrenia; it appears efficacious in treating both sets of symptoms equally well (usual dose range 4 mg o.d.–6 mg o.d for maintenance treatment in adults). Treatment of negative symptoms is mediated by blockade of serotonin $5HT_{2A}$-receptors.
2. Alleviation of affective symptoms associated with schizophrenia – mediated by blockade of serotonin $5HT_{2A}$-receptors.
3. Useful in maintenance treatment of schizophrenic patients – it has been given a licence such that it need only be taken once a day to prevent relapse of schizophrenia.
4. Licensed in the UK in 2004 for the treatment of mania in bipolar disorder:

(i) either as monotherapy or in combination with a mood stabiliser (lithium or valproate), no dose adjustment required.

(i) co-administration with carbamazapine in bipolar mania not recommended.

(ii) usual dose range 1 mg o.d.–6 mg o.d.; continued use must be evaluated and justified on an ongoing basis.

5. Some evidence it may be useful in the treatment of resistant depression – as an augmenting agent to SSRIs (by enhancing serotonergic accumulation within the synapse), although there is no license in this area.

N.B.: *Risperidone is available in the UK as an oral preparation (including a quicklet which may be placed on the tongue or allowed to dissolve or dissolved in water); however IM risperidone, a long-acting intra-muscular injection form of risperidone, was launched in the UK in 2002 (see later under antipsychotic depot injections).*

(c) Adverse effects

1. Less EPSE (at doses up to and including 6 mg o.d.), cf. other antipsychotic drugs; this benefit may be lost at doses of and over 8 mg o.d. – above this dose, it requires twice daily dosing, i.e. the next increment is 5 mg b.d. and this may be gradually increased up to a maximum of 8 mg b.d.
2. Dose dependent elevation in prolactin levels, although these are not necessarily related to the possible sexual side effects.
3. Minimal weight gain due to low affinity for serotonin $5HT_{2c}$-receptors.
4. Postural hypotension – therefore when initiating treatment, the starting dose is 2 mg o.d. on the first day,

which may be increased to 4 mg o.d. on the second day in schizophrenia or to 3 mg o.d. on the second day in bipolar mania; both due to high affinity for α_1-adrenergic receptors.

5. No appreciable anticholinergic side-effects.
6. Side-effects include agitation and insomnia due to possible low affinity for histamine H_1-receptors.
7. Some ECG changes (prolongation of the QT interval). However, there is no requirement for routine ECG monitoring.
8. Not associated with agranulocytosis.
9. Gastrointestinal side-effects – nausea, dyspepsia, abdominal pain.
10. More akathisia, cf. chlorpromazine.

II OLANZAPINE

Introduced into the UK in 1996.

(a) Mode of action

1. Potent dopamine D_2-receptors antagonist; it preferentially blocks D_2-receptors in the mesolimbic cortical bundle, cf. the nigrostriatal pathway.
2. Potent serotonin $5HT_{2A}$-receptors antagonist.
3. High affinity for serotonin $5HT_{2C}$-receptors.
4. Moderate affinity for α_1-adrenergic receptors.
5. High affinity for muscarinic M_1-receptors.
6. High affinity for histamine H_1-receptors.

(b) Indications

1. Treatment of both the positive and negative symptoms of schizophrenia, and affective symptoms associated

with schizophrenia (usual dose 10 mg daily; dose range 5–20 mg for maintenance treatment).

2. Maintenance treatment of schizophrenia (once-per-day dosing).
3. Licensed in the UK in 2003 as monotherapy for the treatment of acute mania (starting dose 15 mg daily) and also for the propyhlaxis of bipolar affective disorder (starting dose 10 mg daily).
4. It may also be used in combination with a mood stabiliser for both the treatment of acute mania and the prophylaxis of bipolar affective disorder (starting dose 10 mg daily).
5. Some evidence it may be useful in the treatment of resistant depression – as an augmenting agent to SSRIs (by enhancing serotonergic accumulation within the synapse), although there is no license in this area.

N.B.: *Olanzapine is available in the UK as an oral preparation, (including a velotab which may be placed on the tongue and allowed to dissolve or dissolved in water); however IM Olanzapine, for use in rapid tranquillisation was launched in the UK in 2004 (see next point).*

6. The rapid tranquillisation of acutely disturbed or violent behaviour in patients with schizophrenia or manic episode, when oral therapy is inappropriate:
   (i) the recommended initial dose of IM olanzapine is 10 mg;
   (ii) a second IM injection, 5–10 mg, may be repeated two hours later;
   (iii) the maximum daily dose of IM olanzapine is 20 mg;
   (iv) the maximum dose of IM olanzapine is 20 mg in 24 hours on 3 consecutive days.

(c) Adverse effects

1. Less EPSE (at doses of 5–10 mg daily), cf. other antipsychotic drugs; this benefit may be lost at doses over 10 mg daily.
2. Sometimes associated with elevation in prolactin level. However, associated clinical manifestations are rare, cf. risperidone.
3. Significant weight gain due to high affinity for serotonin $5HT_{2c}$-receptors; treatment-emergent diabetes mellitus does not appear to be associated with weight gain.
4. Some postural hypotension. However, treatment can be initiated at a therapeutic dose (10 mg daily) without the need to build up from a starting dose; due to moderate affinity for α_1-adrenergic receptors.
5. Anticholinergic side-effects: dry mouth may occur.
6. Side-effects include sedation due to high affinity for histamine H_1-receptors.
7. Some ECG changes (prolongation of the QT interval). However, there is no requirement for routine ECG monitoring.
8. Not associated with agranulocytosis.
9. Some disturbance in LFTs. However, there is no CSM recommendation to monitor LFTs.

III QUETIAPINE

Introduced into the UK in 1997.

(a) Mode of action

1. Weak affinity for dopamine D_2-receptors – similar to clozapine.

2. Low affinity for serotonin $5HT_{2A}$-receptors.
3. Very low affinity for serotonin $5HT_{2C}$-receptors.
4. High affinity for α_1-adrenergic receptors.
5. No appreciable affinity for muscarinic M_1-receptors.
6. High affinity for histamine H_1-receptors.

(b) Indications

1. Treatment of the symptoms of schizophrenia (positive, negative and affective).
2. Maintenance treatment of schizophrenia (twice-per-day dosing; usual dose range 150 mg b.d. to 225 mg b.d. for maintenance treatment).
3. May be effective in the treatment of resistant schizophrenia at higher doses (250 mg b.d. to 375 mg b.d.), i.e. in patients who have failed to respond to another atypical antipsychotic (risperidone, olanzapine).
4. Licensed in the UK in 2003 for the treatment of acute mania either as monotherapy or in combination with a mood stabiliser.

N.B.: *Quetiapine is only currently available in the UK as an oral preparation.*

(c) Adverse effects

1. EPSE comparable with placebo across the dose range (up to, and including, the maximum dose of 375 mg b.d.) – the only atypical antipsychotic currently available in the UK with this feature.
2. Prolactin level comparable with placebo across the dose range (up to, and including, the maximum dose).
3. Minimal weight gain due to very low affinity for serotonin $5HT_{2c}$-receptors.
4. Postural hypotension – therefore when initiating treatment in schizophrenia, the starting dose is 25 mg b.d.,

which is then increased over four days to 150 mg b.d. in adults; it may conveniently be prescribed as a starter pack for the first three days of treatment, and then as 150 mg b.d. from the fourth day onwards; due to high affinity for α_1-adrenergic receptors.

N.B.: *When initiating treatment in acute mania, the starting dose is 50 mg b.d., which is then increased over five days to 300 mg b.d. in adults. The maximum dose for acute mania is 400 mg b.d.*

5. No appreciable anticholinergic side-effects.
6. Side-effects include headaches and somnolence; latter due to high affinity for histamine H_1-receptors.
7. Some ECG changes (prolongation of the QT interval). However, there is no requirement for routine ECG monitoring.
8. Not associated with agranulocytosis, cf. clozapine.
9. Some disturbance in LFTs. However, there is no requirement for the routine monitoring of LFTs.
10. Requires twice daily dosing, cf. risperidone (up to 8 mg daily) and olanzapine which requires once daily dosing; this may reduce compliance in patients taking quetiapine for the long-term treatment of schizophrenia.

IV. AMISULPRIDE

Introduced into the UK in 1997.

(a) Mode of action

1. Blocks dopamine D_3-receptors (mainly presynaptic) and dopamine D_2-receptors (mainly postsynaptic); limbic selective.

2. No affinity for serotonin $5HT_{2A}$-receptors.
3. No affinity for serotonin $5HT_{2C}$-receptors.
4. No affinity for α_1-adrenergic receptors.
5. No affinity for muscarinic M_1-receptors.
6. No affinity for histamine H_1-receptors.

(b) Indications

1. Treatment of schizophrenic patients with florid positive symptoms or a mixture of positive and negative symptoms (usual dose range 200 mg b.d. to 400 mg b.d.; maximum dosage 600 mg b.d.); it can be initiated at 400 mg b.d. for florid positive symptoms.
2. Treatment of schizophrenic patients with predominantly negative symptoms (dose range 50 mg to 300 mg daily with an optimum dosage of 100 mg once a day).

(c) Adverse effects

1. Lower potential for causing EPSE, cf. conventional antipsychotics; however, this benefit is lost at the maximum dosage.
2. Reversible elevation in prolactin level associated with clinical manifestations; not dose dependent and comparable to conventional antipsychotics.
3. Low weight gain due to lack of affinity for serotonin $5HT_{2C}$-receptors.
4. Some postural hypotension. However, treatment can be initiated at a therapeutic dose (200 mg b.d. for positive symptoms with or without negative symptoms) without the need to build up from a starting dose; due to lack of affinity for α_1-adrenergic receptors.
5. No appreciable anticholinergic side-effects.
6. Side-effects include insomnia, anxiety and agitation.

7. Some ECG changes. However, there is no requirement for routine ECG monitoring.
8. Not associated with agranulocytosis, cf. clozapine.
9. There is no requirement for the routine monitoring of LFTs.
10. May be the atypical antipsychotic of choice in patients with diabetes mellitus – due to its lack of affinity for serotonin $5HT_{2C}$-receptors.
11. Requires twice daily dosing, cf. risperidone (up to 8 mg daily) and olanzapinc which require once daily dosing; this may reduce compliance in patients taking amisulpiride for the long term treatment of schizophrenia.

5. ARIPIPRAZOLE

Introduced into the UK in 2004.

(a) Mode of action

1. Partial agonist at dopamine D_2-receptors:
   (i) Acts as a dopamine D_2-receptor agonist on presynaptic autoreceptors.
   (ii) Acts as a dopamine D_2-receptor antagonist on postsynaptic receptors.
   (iii) Apripiprazole acts as a dopamine system stabiliser in both hypodopaminergic and hyperdopaminergic conditions. As shown in animal models *in vivo*, stabilisation of the dopamine system is proposed to provide antipsychotic efficacy with minimal adverse effects.
2. Partial agonist at serotonin $5HT_{1A}$-receptors.
   (i) May protect against dopamine-mediated adverse effects.

(ii) May provide anxiolytic activity.

3. High affinity for serotonin $5HT_{2A}$-receptors.
4. Low affinity for serotonin $5HT_{2C}$-receptors.
5. Low affinity for α_1-adrenergic receptors.
6. Low affinity for muscarinic M_1-receptors.
7. Low affinity for histamine H_1-receptors.

(b) Indications

1. Treatment of the positive symptoms of schizophrenia – due to its action as a dopamine D_2-receptor antagonist in the mesolimbic area (where dopamine is excessive).
2. Treatment of the negative symptoms of schizophrenia – due to its action as a dopamine D_2-receptor agonist in the mesocortical area (where dopamine is deficient).

N.B.: *The dosing is 15–30 mg once daily.*

(c) Adverse effects

1. EPSE comparable with placebo.
2. Prolactin level comparable with placebo.
3. Minimum weight gain due to lack of affinity for $5HT_{2C}$ serotonin receptors.
4. Some postural hypotension. However, treatment can be initiated at a therapeutic dose (15 mg) without the need to build up from a starting dose; due to low affinity for α_1-adrenergic receptors.
5. No appreciable anticholinergic side-effects.
6. Side-effects include akathisia and the risk of seizures.
7. Not associated with ECG changes – therefore no requirement for routine ECG monitoring.
8. Not associated with agranulocytosis, cf. clozapine.
9. No requirement for the routine monitoring of LFTs.
10. No dose adjustments required in those with renal or hepatic impairment.

6. ZOTEPINE

Introduced into the UK in 1998.

(a) Mode of action

1. Moderate affinity for dopamine D_2-receptors
2. High affinity for serotonin $5HT_{2A}$-receptors.
3. High affinity for serotonin $5HT_{2C}$-receptors.
4. Low affinity for α_1-adrenergic receptors.
5. Potent noradrenaline reuptake inhibitor.
6. Low affinity for muscarinic M_1-receptors.
7. High affinity for histamine H_1-receptors.

(b) Indications

1. Treatment of the symptoms of schizophrenia – it has a general license for this, i.e. it is not specifically licensed for any individual set of symptoms, (positive, negative or affective). However, it may have antidepressant effects due to its action as a potent noradrenaline reuptake inhibitor.
2. It is initiated in adults at the therapeutic dose of 25 mg t.d.s.; if further clinical improvement is required this may be increased to 50 mg t.d.s.; it may be further increased to a maximum of 100 mg t.d.s. if required.

N.B.: *Zotepine is only currently available in the UK as an oral preparation.*

(c) Adverse effects

1. May have lower potential for causing EPSE, cf conventional antipsychotics.
2. Sometimes associated with elevation in prolactin levels. However, associated clinical manifestations are rare.

3. Significant weight gain due to high affinity for serotonin $5HT_{2C}$-receptors.
4. Some postural hypotension. However, treatment can be initiated at a therapeutic dose without the need to build up from a starting dose; due to low affinity for α_1-adrenergic receptors.
5. Dry mouth due to potent noradrenaline reuptake inhibition.
6. Side-effects include sedation due to high affinity for histamine H_1-receptors.
7. Other side-effects include aesthenia, constipation, tachycardia and seizures.
8. ECG changes (prolongation of the QT interval) associated with a possible increased risk of toxicity. In view of this, CSM recommends an ECG prior to commencing treatment in patients at risk of arrythmias. Zotepine should therefore be used with caution in patients with clinically significant cardiac disease.
9. Sometimes associated with neutropenia. Therefore if an infection occurs, a full blood count should be checked.
10. Sometimes associated with elevation in transaminases. Therefore in patients with known hepatic impairment, liver function tests should be monitored weekly for the first three months.
11. Zotepine is uricosuric, therefore it should not be started within three weeks of resolution of an episode of acute gout.
12. Requires dosing three times a day, cf risperidone (up to 8 mg daily) and olanzapine which require once daily dosing; this may reduce compliance in patients taking zotepine for the long-term treatment of schizophrenia.

VII. CLOZAPINE

(a) Mode of action

1. Moderate affinity for dopamine D_2-receptors.
2. More active at dopamine D_4-receptors, cf. other antipsychotics.
3. High affinity for serotonin $5HT_{2A}$-receptors.
4. High affinity for serotonin $5HT_{2C}$-receptors.
5. High affinity for α_1-adrenergic receptors.
6. High affinity for muscarinic M_1-receptors.
7. High affinity for muscarinic M_4-receptors.
8. High affinity for histamine H_1-receptors.

(b) Indications

The treatment of schizophrenia in patients unresponsive to, or intolerant of, conventional antipsychotic drugs; at least one drug from two chemically distinct classes should be given a full therapeutic trial before considering clozapine (the atypical antipsychotics may be used as first line treatment of schizophrenia); in addition, it may be worth considering a course of electroconvulsive therapy (ECT) before starting clozapine therapy, since this can be an effective treatment in resistant schizophrenia (particularly when a significant affective component is present).
N.B.: *Clozapine treatment must only be instituted by psychiatrists registered with the Clozaril Patient Monitoring Service (CPMS).*

(c) Adverse effects

1. Less EPSE, cf. conventional antipsychotics.
2. Asymptomatic rise in serum prolactin.
3. Significant weight gain due to high affinity for serotonin $5HT_{2C}$-receptors; treatment-emergent diabetes

mellitus does not appear to be associated with weight gain.

4. Postural hypotension with risk of collapse – therefore treatment should be initiated with a starting dose and then gradually increased over 14–21 days to 300 mg daily in divided doses; usual dose 200–450 mg daily (max. 900 mg daily).
5. Anticholinergic side-effects: hypersalivation due to high affinity for muscarinic M_4-receptors in the salivary glands is common; other atropinic side-effects due to muscarinic M_1-receptor blockade also occur.
6. Side-effects include sedation due to high affinity for histamine H_1-receptors.
7. Other side-effects include fits and rare instances of myocarditis.
8. Some ECG changes. However, there is no requirement for routine ECG monitoring.
9. It causes agranulocytosis (life-threatening) in 2–3% of patients taking the drug – its use is therefore restricted to patients registered with the clozaril patient monitoring service (CPMS) whereby the patient has regular full blood counts to detect any possible agranulocytosis; should this occur, the clozapine must be stopped.
10. No requirement for the routine monitoring of LFTs.
11. Requires twice daily dosing, cf. risperidone (up to 8 mg daily) and olanzapine which require once daily dosing; this may reduce complicance in patients taking clozapine for the long term treatment of schizophrenia (as may the requirement for regular full blood counts).

ANTIPSYCHOTIC DEPOT INJECTIONS

A. IN GENERAL

(a) Mode of action

Long-acting depot injections administered intramuscularly as an oily injection and slowly released into the bloodstream.

(b) Indications

1. For maintenance therapy of schizophrenia – more conveniently given than oral antipsychotic preparations ensuring better patient compliance.
2. For prophylaxis of bipolar affective disorder in patients who have poor compliance with oral prophylactic medication (mood stabilisers) – depot medication certainly protects against hypomanic relapse and some clinicians believe it also protects against a subsequent depressive relapse.

(c) Adverse effects

1. Initially patients should always be given a test dose injection to ensure that the patient does not experience undue side-effects or any idiosyncratic reactions to the medication or formulation.
2. They may give rise to a higher incidence of EPSE – cf. oral antipsychotic preparations.

B. MORE SPECIFICALLY

1. Fluphenazine decanoate

(a) Indications

1. Useful in treating agitated or aggressive schizophrenic patients.
2. May be useful for the control of aggressive patients (in view of its sedative nature).

(b) Adverse effect

Contraindicated in severely depressed states – in view of its tendency to cause depression.

2. Flupenthixol decanoate

(a) Indication

Useful in treating retarded or withdrawn schizophrenic patients – in view of its apparent alerting nature.

(b) Adverse effect

Not suitable for the treatment of agitated or aggressive schizophrenic patients – since it can cause over-excitement in such patients in view of its alerting nature.

3. Zuclopenthixol decanoate

(a) Indications

1. Useful in treating agitated or aggressive schizophrenic patients.
2. May be useful for the control of aggressive patients (this specific indication is more clearly established for

zuclopenthixol decanoate – cf. fluphenazine decanoate) – in view of its sedative nature (zuclopenthixol decanoate is more sedative than fluphenazine decanoate).

(b) Adverse effect

Not suitable for the treatment of retarded or withdrawn schizophrenic patients – since it may exacerbate psychomotor retardation in such patients in view of its sedative nature.

4. Haloperidol Decanoate

(a) Indication

Maintenance in schizophrenia and other psychosis; usually 4-weekly administration.

5. Pipothiazine Palmitate

(a) Indication

Maintenance in schizophrenia and other psychosis; 4-weekly administration.

(b) Adverse effect

Allegedly lower EPSE, cf. other conventional antipsychotic depot injections.

6. IM Risperidone

(a) Indication

1. The world's first ever atypical antipsychotic long-acting intramuscular injection – launched in the UK in 2002.

2. Licensed for the treatment of both the positive and negative symptoms of schizophrenia; it also alleviates affective symptoms associated with schizophrenia; 2-weekly administration.
3. May be the 'depot' (long-acting intramuscular injection) of choice in patients with bipolar affective disorder who are poorly compliant with oral mood stabilisers.

(b) Adverse effect

Less EPSE, cf. other conventional antipsychotic depot injections.

CHAPTER 3

Antidepressant Drugs

CLASSIFICATION

Tricyclic Antidepressants (TCAs)

1. Amitriptyline
2. Imipramine
3. Dothiepin
4. Trazodone
5. Clomipramine

Monoamine Oxidase Inhibitors (MAOIs)

Reversible Inhibitors of Monoamine Oxidase Type (RIMAs)

Second Generation Antidepressants

1. Lofepramine
2. Mianserin

Selective Serotonin Reuptake Inhibitors (SSRIs)

1. Fluvoxamine
2. Fluoxetine
3. Sertraline
4. Paroxetine
5. Citalopram
6. Escitalopram

Serotonin and noradrenaline reuptake inhibitors (SNRIs)

Noradrenergic and specific serotonergic antidepressants (NaSSAs)

Noradrenaline reuptake inhibitors (NARIs)

1. Pindolol
2. Thyroxine

I. TRICYCLIC ANTIDEPRESSANTS (TCAs)

A. IN GENERAL

(a) Mode of action

Monoamine reuptake inhibitors (MARIs) – inhibit the reuptake of both serotonin and noradrenaline into the presynaptic neurone, with the result that both neurotransmitters accumulate within the synapse. Such biochemical changes occur within several hours following administration of the drug, while the antidepressant action of the drug is delayed for about 2 weeks, indicating that some secondary process must be taking place.

(b) Indications

I. Affective disorders:
   A. Treatment of depressive disorders in the acute stage.
   B. Preventing relapse of depressive disorders – need to continue medication for 6 months postclinical recovery after the first episode of a unipolar affective disorder and for several (1–3) years

postclinical recovery after 2 or more episodes of a unipolar affective disorder.

N.B.: (i) *If the first episode of the depressive disorder is totally destructive to the patient's life, lifelong antidepressant medication should be considered postclinical recovery, as patients cannot afford to have relapses of their disorders.*

(ii) *For the last decade or so, the generally held view among informed psychiatrists has been that 'the dose that gets you well is the dose that keeps you well'.*

(iii) *TCAs are safer to use in pregnancy where the effects are more clearly established, cf. the more recently introduced antidepressants (SSRIs, SNRIs, NaSSAs and NARIs).*

(iv) *Antidepressants are non-addictive but are associated with a discontinuation syndrome – therefore they should be gradually withdrawn over a period of 4 weeks (when on the maximum dose), to minimise the risk of discontinuation symptoms.*

II. Anxiety disorders (generalised anxiety disorder and panic disorder) – when medication has to be prolonged beyond the few (2–4) weeks for which benzodiazepines are prescribed; effective due to their anxiolytic properties.

III. Phobic anxiety disorders – again effective due to their anxiolytic properties.

IV. Obsessive compulsive disorders – when anxiolytic treatment has to be prolonged beyond the few (2–4) weeks for which benzodiazepines are prescribed.

N.B.: *Clomipramine is claimed to have a specific anti-obsessional effect in addition to its anxiolytic effect (see later).*

V. Hypochondriasis – some clinicians advocate a trial of TCAs in all patients (especially if the patient is depressed).

VI. Chronic organic disorder with depressive symptoms – a trial of antidepressant medication is worthwhile even in the presence of dementia.

N.B.: *TCAs tend to increase confusion in the elderly due to anticholinergic side-effects – therefore SSRIs and SNRIs are the preferred antidepressants.*

VII. Bulimia nervosa – TCAs produce an immediate reduction in binging and vomiting. However, their long-term effects are less pronounced.

(c) Side-effects

1. Anticholinergic side-effects:
   - (i) Dry mouth.
   - (ii) Blurred vision.
   - (iii) Constipation.
   - (iv) Urinary retention.
   - (v) Tachycardia.
   - (vi) Impotence.
   - (vii) Sweating.
   - (viii) Confusion.
   - (ix) Exacerbation of narrow angle glaucoma.
2. Cardiovascular side-effects (due to quinidine-like actions):
   - (i) Tachycardia.
   - (ii) Arrhythmias.
   - (iii) Postural hypotension.
   - (iv) Syncope.
   - (v) Cardiomyopathy.
   - (vi) Cardiac failure.
   - (vii) ECG changes (e.g. inversion and flattening of T

waves).

3. Other side-effects:
   - (i) Seizures (due to lowering of the convulsive threshold).
   - (ii) Hypomania (in patients with bipolar affective disorder).
   - (iii) Tremor.
   - (iv) Weight gain.
   - (v) Agranulocytosis (uncommon).
   - (vi) NMS (rare).
   - (vii) Tardive dyskinesia (rare).

(d) Toxic effects (i.e. effects of overdosage)

1. Cardiac arrhythmias/arrest.
2. Prolongation of the QT interval.
3. Postural hypotension.
4. Epileptic seizures.
5. Hyperreflexia.
6. Mydriasis.
7. Coma.
8. Death.

B. MORE SPECIFICALLY

1. Amitriptyline

(a) Indications

Treatment of agitated depression – in view of its sedative nature:

1. Starting dose – 75 mg nocte; build up gradually over 1–2 weeks to 150 mg nocte (usual dose required for efficacy in treating both the acute stage and for prophylaxis).
2. In patients unresponsive to 150 mg nocte – pushing the

dose up to 225 mg nocte or even 300 mg nocte (maximum) may be clinically effective; this would require ECG monitoring, as it is above the BNF maximum recommended dose (200 mg nocte).

(b) Adverse effects

Less suitable for the treatment of retarded depression – since it may exacerbate psychomotor retardation in such patients in view of its sedative nature.

2. Imipramine

(a) Indications

1. Treatment of retarded depression – in view of its alerting nature (similar dosage requirements as for amitriptyline – see earlier).
2. Treatment of anxiety disorders – imipramine may have a specific effect on autonomic reactivity in panic disorder (where the starting dose is 25 mg).
3. Treatment of phobic anxiety disorders – some clinicians consider imipramine to be the treatment of choice in agoraphobia.

(b) Adverse effects

Less suitable for the treatment of agitated depression – since it may cause over-excitement in such patients in view of its alerting nature.

3. Dothiepin

(a) Indication

Treatment of agitated depression – in view of its sedative nature:

1. Starting dose – 75 mg nocte, increased after 4 days to 150 mg nocte.
2. In patients unresponsive to 150 mg nocte – pushing the dose up to 225 mg nocte may be clinically effective.
3. Particularly useful in treating elderly patients – since it has less anticholinergic side-effects and less cardiovascular side-effects – cf. amitriptyline (this also explains why the starting dose of dothiepin can be stepped up more quickly to the therapeutic dose – cf. amitriptyline).

(b) Adverse effect

If taken in overdosage, dothiepin is the TCA most commonly responsible for deaths in the UK at present.

4. Trazodone

(a) Mode of action

An antidepressant drug related to the TCAs – but a more selective inhibitor of the reuptake of serotonin, cf. amitriptyline and imipramine.

(b) Indication

1. Treatment of depression with associated anxiety – in view of its sedative nature:
   (i) Starting dose – 150 mg nocte.
   (ii) May be increased to 300 mg daily.
   (iii) Maximum dose of 600 mg daily in divided doses in hospitalised patients (in adults).
2. Very useful in the elderly in the treatment of dementia associated with agitation and aggression – usually up to 300 mg daily.

(c) Adverse effects

1. Less anticholinergic side-effects and less cardiovascular side-effects, cf. amitriptyline.
2. Safer in overdosage, cf. dothiepin.
3. Rarely priapism (discontinue immediately).

5. Clomipramine

(a) Mode of action

Inhibits the reuptake of both serotonin and noradrenaline. However, it is a more selective inhibitor of the reuptake of serotonin, cf. the other TCAs.

(b) Indications

1. Treatment of agitated depression – in view of its sedative nature.
2. Treatment of obsessive compulsive disorder – it has been reported that clomipramine has a specific action against obsessional symptoms (owing to its being a more selective reuptake inhibitor of serotonin, cf. the other TCAs).
3. Treatment of panic disorder – it has been reported that clomipramine in low doses has a specific action against panic symptoms (owing to its being a more selective reuptake inhibitor of serotonin, cf. the other TCAs).

(c) Side-effects

It has more anticholinergic side-effects and more cardiovascular side-effects – cf. amitriptyline – which may prevent some patients from tolerating it.

II. MONOAMINE OXIDASE INHIBITORS (MAOIs)

(a) Mode of action

Inhibit the enzyme monoamine oxidase which is present in the presynaptic neurone and provides an important pathway for the metabolism of monoamines; thus, MAOIs inhibit the intraneuronal metabolism of monoamines, resulting in enhanced release of amine neurotransmitters into the synapse.

(b) Indications

1. Treatment of atypical depressive disorders with anxiety, phobic anxiety or obsessional symptoms (i.e. neurotic symptoms).
2. Treatment of resistant depression (particularly tranylcypromine – but it carries a risk of dependence because of its amphetamine-like action).
3. Treatment of anxiety disorders – some evidence for usefulness in panic disorders owing to anxiolytic properties.
4. Treatment of phobic anxiety disorders – reduce agoraphobic symptoms, but there is a high relapse rate when drugs are stopped.

(c) Adverse effects

1. Potentiate the pressor effect of tyramine and dopa present in certain foods (e.g. Chianti wine, cheese spreads, well-hung game, pickled herring, banana skins, broad bean 'pods', Marmite and Bovril).
2. Potentiate the pressor effect of indirect-acting sympathomimetic drugs (e.g. proprietary cough mixtures,

nasal decongestants, anaesthetics).

N.B.: *Both of these types of interaction may cause a dangerous rise in blood pressure ('hypertensive crisis') with fatal consequences; an early warning sign may be a throbbing headache.*

3. TCAs, second-generation antidepressants and SSRIs should not be started until 2 weeks after MAOIs have been stopped in view of the persistence of the effects of MAOIs following discontinuation.
4. MAOIs should not be started until 1 week after TCAs and second-generation antidepressants have been stopped.
5. MAOIs should not be started until 2 weeks after SSRIs have been stopped with the exception of fluoxetine (see below).
6. MAOIs should not be started until 5 weeks after fluoxetine has been stopped in view of its long half-life and active metabolite (norfluoxetine).
7. The most commonly prescribed MAOI is phenelzine; however, MAOIs are the least commonly prescribed of the antidepressant drugs because:
   (i) They interact dangerously with certain foods and drugs (see above).
   (ii) The washout period following MAOI discontinuation is 2 weeks – cf. the washout period of 1 week following discontinuation of TCAs and second-generation antidepressants (see above).
   (iii) The main indication for MAOIs is atypical depressive disorders (see above), i.e. MAOIs are not generally indicated for endogenous depressive disorders with biological features of depression (except resistant cases when they may be combined with TCAs under specialist supervision).

III. REVERSIBLE INHIBITORS OF MONOAMINE OXIDASE TYPE A (RIMAs)

Moclobemide (the first RIMA) was introduced into the UK in 1993.

(a) Mode of action

Selectively and reversibly inhibits monoamine oxidase type A. In contrast, conventional MAOIs inhibit monoamine oxidase types A and B and are irreversible.

The antidepressant effect of MAOIs is considered to be a result of inhibition of monoamine oxidase type A.

(b) Indications

1. Treatment of endogenous and atypical depressive disorders (dosage: 150–600 mg daily in divided doses; however, there are anecdotal reports of higher doses required for efficacy in endogenous depressive disorders).
2. Treatment of resistant depression (particularly when the patient is unwilling to try a conventional MAOI).
3. Treatment of anxiety disorders and phobic anxiety disorders (particularly social phobias).

(c) Adverse effects

1. Claimed to cause less potentiation of the pressor effect of tyramine and dopa-containing foods, cf. conventional MAOIs – however, patients should still avoid consuming large amounts of such foods.
2. Claimed to cause less potentiation of the pressor effect of indirect-acting sympathomimetic drugs, cf. con-

ventional MAOIs – however, patients should still avoid such drugs.

3. No treatment-free washout period is required after it has been stopped in view of its short duration of action, cf. conventional MAOIs.
4. Should not be started until 1 week after TCAs, second-generation antidepressants and conventional MAOIs have been stopped.
5. Should not be started until 2 weeks after SSRIs have been stopped with the exception of fluoxetine (see below).
6. Should not be started until 5 weeks after fluoxetine has been stopped.
7. Contraindicated in agitated or excited patients – an unfortunate adverse effect since the majority of clinically depressed patients present this way.
8. May precipitate hypomania in patients with bipolar affective disorder.
9. May be the antidepressant of choice in patients with epilepsy.

IV. SECOND-GENERATION ANTI-DEPRESSANTS

A. IN GENERAL

(a) Definition

The next class of antidepressant drugs to be developed after TCAs.

(b) Indications

Particularly useful in the following groups of depressed patients:

1. Patients intolerant of the side-effects of TCAs.
2. Elderly patients.
3. Patients at high risk of suicide.
4. Patients treated in the general practice setting.

(c) Adverse effects

1. Less anticholinergic side-effects and less cardiovascular side-effects – cf. TCAs.
2. Safer in overdosage – cf. TCAs.

B. MORE SPECIFICALLY

1. Lofepramine

(a) Mode of action

1. Mainly a noradrenergic reuptake inhibitor, i.e. it is a relatively selective reuptake inhibitor of noradrenaline.
2. Structurally a tricyclic antidepressant – however, its adverse effects profile is considerably different from the older 'parent' TCAs (see below).

(b) Indication

Treatment and prophylaxis of retarded depression – in view of its alerting nature (dosage: 70 mg b.d.; this may be increased to 70 mg mane, 140 mg nocte).

(c) Adverse effects

1. Less suitable for the treatment of agitated depression – since it may cause over-excitement (e.g. sweating, pal-

pitations) in such patients in view of its alerting nature.

2. Much improved side-effects profile – cf. older 'parent' TCAs – i.e. lofepramine has fewer anticholinergic side-effects and less cardiotoxicity. Hence, more suitable for use in physically ill patients, cf. older 'parent' TCAs.
3. Remarkable record of safety in overdosage – only three deaths recorded to date.
4. May be the antidepressant of choice in pregnancy.

2. Mianserin

(a) Mode of action

1. An α_2-presynaptic autoreceptor antagonist – a novel mode of action for an antidepressant drug with no significant effect on the reuptake of monoamines (i.e. it is only a weak inhibitor of serotonin and noradrenaline reuptake); despite this, it still appears to be an effective antidepressant.
2. Structurally a tetracyclic antidepressant.

(b) Adverse effects

1. No anticholinergic side-effects.
2. Minimal cardiotoxicity – safer in overdosage.
3. Rarely causes convulsions – i.e. less proconvulsive.

(items 1–3: cf. TCAs)

4. May cause agranulocytosis (particularly in the elderly):
   (i) A full blood count is recommended every 4 weeks during the first 3 months of treatment.
   (ii) If signs of infection develop (e.g. sore throat, fever, stomatitis), treatment should be stopped, a full blood count obtained and subsequent clinical monitoring should continue.

(iii) This unfortunate side-effect of mianserin together with its questionable efficacy (see mode of action earlier) has limited the prescription of the drug in the hospital setting.

V. SELECTIVE SEROTONIN REUPTAKE INHIBITORS (SSRIs) (ALSO KNOWN AS 5HT REUPTAKE INHIBITORS)

A. IN GENERAL

(a) Definition

The next class of antidepressant drugs to follow the second-generation antidepressants in time, i.e. SSRIs, are effectively 'third-generation antidepressants'.

(b) Mode of action

SSRIs are highly selective serotonin reuptake inhibitors with little or no effect on noradrenergic processes.

(c) Indications

1. Treatment of depressive disorders, particularly in:
   (i) Patients intolerant of the side-effects of TCAs.
   (ii) Elderly patients.
   (iii) Patients with a high risk of suicide.
   (iv) Patients treated in the general practice setting.
   (v) Patients with cardiovascular disease.
2. Preventing relapse of depressive disorders – need to continue medication for 6 months postclinical recovery after the first episode of a unipolar affective disorder

and for several (1–3) years postclinical recovery after 2 or more episodes of a unipolar affective disorder.

N.B.: *If the patient fails to respond to one SSRI after an adequate trial (i.e. 4–6 weeks at the maximum dose), there is a tendency to try one other SSRI before switching to a different class of antidepressant.*

3. Treatment of panic disorder.
4. Treatment of obsessive compulsive disorder.
5. Treatment of bulimia nervosa.
6. Treatment of post-traumatic stress disorder (PTSD).
7. Treatment of social anxiety disorder (social phobia).
8. Treatment of generalised anxiety disorder (GAD).
9. Treatment of aggressive behaviour.*
10. Treatment of alcohol dependence – there is some evidence that SSRIs reduce alcohol craving and alcohol consumption in patients with this syndrome.*

(d) Adverse effects

1. No anticholinergic side-effects.
2. No clinically significant cardiovascular side-effects.
3. Safer in overdosage.
4. More gastrointestinal side-effects (e.g. nausea, vomiting, diarrhoea) which are dose related.
5. More sexual dysfunction (e.g. delayed ejaculation in men, anorgasmia in women).

(Items 1–5: cf. TCA)

6. In keeping with good clinical practice, SSRIs should be withdrawn slowly to minimise the risk of discontinuation symptoms.
7. Inhibition of the liver enzyme cytochrome P4502D6, which is responsible for metabolizing the SSRIs and other drugs that might be coprescribed. There is little

*These two indications are not currently licensed in the UK.

convincing evidence of clinically significant drug interactions.

8. No clinically significant interaction with alcohol – therefore SSRIs may be prescribed to patients co-morbid for alcohol problems and clinical depression.
9. May be less likely to precipitate hypomania in patients with bipolar affective disorder, cf. TCAs.
10. May only be prescribed at a therapeutic dose, cf. TCAs which have tended to be prescribed at a subtherapeutic dose in the general practice setting.
11. Less likely to cause weight gain, cf. TCAs.
12. EPSE (including akathisia) are reported to the CSM.

B. MORE SPECIFICALLY

1. Fluvoxamine

The first SSRI introduced into the UK in 1987.

(a) Mode of action

1. Structurally a monocyclic antidepressant.
2. No active metabolite.
3. 17–22 hour half-life.

(b) Indications

1. Treatment of depression (dosage: 50 mg b.d.–150 mg b.d.).
2. Treatment of obsessive compulsive disorder (dosage: 50 mg b.d.–150 mg b.d.).

(c) Adverse effects

1. High incidence of nausea and vomiting particularly during the first few days of treatment – this may

prevent some patients from tolerating it; such gastro-intestinal side-effects may be offset somewhat by taking tablets immediately after food and by initiating treatment at a dosage of 50 mg nocte for 1 week and then stepping it up to the usual therapeutic dosage of 50 mg b.d. (some patients may only respond to the higher therapeutic dosage of 100 mg b.d. or the even higher dosage of 150 mg b.d.).

2. Less suitable for patients with hepatic impairment – since it may elevate hepatic enzymes with symptoms.
3. Increases the plasma concentration of theophylline.

2. Fluoxetine

Introduced into the UK in 1989.

(a) Mode of action

1. Structurally a bicyclic antidepressant.
2. Long half-life (2–4 days) with an active metabolite (norfluoxetine) which itself has a long half-life with similar activity to the parent compound.

(b) Indications

1. Treatment of depression (dosage: 20 mg mane).
2. Treatment of bulimia nervosa (dosage: 60 mg mane).
3. Treatment of obsessive compulsive disorder – dose range: 20–60 mg mane; increasing the dosage within this range increasingly targets obsessional symptoms.

(c) Adverse effects

1. Less suitable for patients with severe renal impairment – in view of its long half-life and active metabolite.
2. Less suitable for patients with severe weight loss – in

view of its catabolic/anorectic nature.

3. Nausea and vomiting appear to be less of a problem with fluoxetine, cf. fluvoxamine.
4. Increases the plasma concentration of the antiarrhythmic flecainide by cytochrome P4502D6 inhibition.
5. Other significant drug interactions – increases the plasma concentration of:
   (i) Haloperidol
   (ii) Clozapine
   (iii) TCAs
   (iv) Phenytoin
   (v) Warfarin

3. Sertraline

Introduced into the UK in 1990.

(a) Mode of action

1. Structurally different from fluvoxamine, fluoxetine and paroxetine.
2. Has an active metabolite (desmethylsertraline) which has a long half-life with about one eighth of the activity of the parent compound.

(b) Indications

1. Treatment of depression (dose range: 50 mg mane to 200 mg mane).
2. Prevention of relapse in depression and recurrent depression.
3. Treatment of obsessive compulsive disorder (dose range: 50 mg mane to 200 mg mane).
4. Treatment of post-traumatic stress disorder in women only (starting dose 25 mg mane for one week; dose

range: 50 mg mane to 200 mg mane).

(c) Adverse effects

1. Side-effects include loose stools and diarrhoea.
2. May have lower potential for drug interactions – since it has no significant interaction with cytochrome P4502D6.

4. Paroxetine

Introduced into the UK in 1991.

(a) Mode of action

1. Structurally different from fluvoxamine, fluoxetine and sertraline.
2. No active metabolite.
3. 24-hour half-life.

(b) Indications

1. Treatment of depression with associated anxiety – the first SSRI to have a licence for this (dosage: 20 mg mane; this may be increased up to 50 mg daily in adults by gradual 10 mg increments if necessary).
2. Treatment of obsessive compulsive disorder (OCD) (dosage: 20 mg mane; this may be increased up to 60 mg daily in adults by weekly 10 mg increments if necessary). It may be the SSRI of choice to treat OCD, owing to its established anxiolytic profile and anti-obsessional effect.
3. The first SSRI to have a licence for the treatment of panic disorder (dosage: 10 mg mane; this may be increased up to 50 mg daily in adults by weekly 10 mg increments if necessary).

4. Prevention of relapse in depression.
5. Prevention of relapse in obsessive compulsive disorder (OCD).
6. Prevention of relapse in panic disorder.
7. Treatment of social anxiety disorder (social phobia) (dosage: 20 mg mane; if no improvement after at least two weeks, this may be increased up to 50 mg daily in adults by weekly 10 mg increments is necessary).
8. The first SSRI to have a license for the treatment of post-traumatic stress disorder (PTSD) (dosage: 20 mg mane; this may be increased up to 50 mg daily in adults by gradual 10 mg increments if necessary).
9. Treatment of generalised anxiety disorder (GAD) (dosage: 20 mg mane in UK; 20 mg–50 mg mane in USA).

(c) Adverse effects

1. Less suitable for the treatment of retarded (anergic) depression – in view of its anxiolytic nature.
2. Nausea and vomiting appear to be less of a problem with paroxetine, cf. fluvoxamine.
3. Inhibits its own metabolism by cytochrome P4502D6 inhibition.
4. Side-effects include a dry mouth and drowsiness.
5. During the initial treatment of panic disorder, there is potential for a worsening of the panic symptoms (hence the starting dose is 10 mg mane, cf. 20 mg mane for other indications).
6. When discontinuing Paroxetine, it should be gradually reduced by weekly 10 mg increments to minimise the risk of discontinuation symptoms, i.e. when on the maximum dose of 50 mg daily in adults for depression, this should be gradually withdrawn over a period of 4 weeks.

5. Citalopram

Introduced into the UK in 1995.

(a) Mode of action

1. Structurally different from the other SSRIs.
2. No active metabolite.

(b) Indications

1. Treatment of depression (dosage: 20 mg daily; this may be increased up to 60 mg daily in adults by gradual 20 mg increments if necessary).
2. Prevention of relapse in depression and recurrent depression.
3. Treatment of panic disorder (dosage: 10 mg daily; this may be increased up to 60 mg daily in adults by weekly 10 mg increments if necessary; however, the usual recommended dose is 20–30 mg daily).

(c) Adverse effects

1. May have lower potential for drug interactions – since it has no significant interaction with cytochrome P4502D6.

6. Escitalopram

Introduced into the UK in 2002.

(a) Mode of action

1. The *S*-enantiomer of citalopram, i.e. the optical isomer of citalopram with antidepressant activity.
2. More selective than citalopram – which consists of the racemic mixture of both the *S*-enantiomer and

the *R*-enantiomer (the latter lacks antidepressant activity).

3. Serotonin transporter theory:
   (i) By removing *R*-citalopram (at the synapse), escitalopram functions more effectively.
   (ii) Escitalopram increases serotonin levels more than citalopram.

(b) Indications

1. Treatment of depression (dosage: 10 mg daily; this may be increased up to 20 mg daily in adults).
2. Treatment of panic disorder with or without agoraphobia (starting dose 5 mg daily for one week; dosage: 10–20 mg daily).
3. Licensed for treatment of social anxiety disorder in 2004 (ususal dosage 10 mg daily; dose range 5–20 mg daily).
4. May be associated with an early symptom relief.
5. Some evidence that efficacy is comparable to venlafaxine XL, cf. other SSRIs where there is considerable evidence that venlafaxine XL is more effective.

(c) Adverse effects

1. Escitalopram has a comparable side-effect profile to citalopram.
2. Co-administration with the known cytochrome P450 isoenzyme CYP2C19 inhibitors omeprazole and high dose cimetidine, may require reduction of the escitalopram dose (metabolism of escitalopram is mainly mediated by CYP2C19).

VI. SEROTONIN AND NORADRENALINE REUPTAKE INHIBITORS (SNRIs)

Venlafaxine (the first SNRI) was introduced into the UK in 1995.

Available as a standard formulation requiring twice daily dosing (up to 375 mg daily) and a modified release formulation (XL) to allow once daily dosing (up to 225 mg daily)

(a) Mode of action

1. Structurally a bicyclic antidepressant.
2. It selectively inhibits the reuptake of both serotonin and noradrenaline into the presynaptic neurone (but the predominant effect is on serotonin).
   (i) at low dose (75 mg daily) – its predominant action (80%) is on serotonin inhibition, with a lesser action (20%) on noradrenaline inhibition.
   (ii) at moderate dose to high dose – it acts more equally as both a serotonin and noradrenaline reuptake inhibitor.

(b) Indication

1. Treatment of depressive disorders (dosage: 75 mg daily; this may be increased to 150 mg daily in mild to moderate depression and again if necessary to the maximum dose of 225 mg daily for the XL formulation; it may be further increased by 75 mg increments every 2–3 days to a maximum of 375 mg daily in hospitalized severe depression – this would require twice daily dosing of the standard formulation.
2. There is now considerable evidence that venlafaxine

XL is more effective than the SSRIs; however, there is some evidence that the efficacy of escitalopram is comparable to venlafaxine XL.

3. Treatment of generalised anxiety disorder (GAD) (dosage: 75 mg daily in UK; 75 mg–225 mg daily in USA).

(c) Adverse effects

1. Less anticholinergic side effects. } cf. TCAs
2. Less clinically significant cardiovascular side-effects. } cf. TCAs
3. Safer in overdosage. } cf. TCAs
4. Less likely to cause weight gain. } cf. TCAs
5. Gastrointestinal side-effects (e.g. nausea) – these are dose related and occur with a similar prevalence to those observed with SSRIs; they appear to be reduced with the XL formulation.
6. Blood pressure should be monitored in patients taking 75 mg daily or more.
7. May precipitate hypomania in patients with bipolar affective disorder.
8. Frequently reported side-effects are sweating and headache.
9. Drug interactions – potentiation of the anticoagulant effects of warfarin have been reported.

VII. NORADRENERGIC AND SPECIFIC SEROTONERGIC ANTIDEPRESSANTS (NaSSAs)

Mirtazapine (the first NaSSA) was launched in the UK in 1997 as a conventional tablet. This was phased out by 4th

May 2004.

The world's first ever antidepressant available as an orally disintegrating tablet – launched in the UK in 2003. This soltab formulation should be placed on the tongue and allowed to dissolve, i.e. melt.

(a) Mode of action

1. A presynaptic α_2-autoreceptor antagonist – thus enhancing noradrenergic neurotransmission (like mianserin).
2. A presynaptic α_2-heteroreceptor antagonist – thus preventing the inhibitory effect of noradrenaline on serotonin receptors.
3. A postsynaptic serotonin $5HT_2$- and $5HT_3$-receptor antagonist – thus enhancing serotonergic neurotransmission specifically via serotonin $5HT_1$-postsynaptic receptors.
4. No significant effect on the reuptake of monoamines, cf. TCAs, SSRIs and SNRIs.
5. A postsynaptic histamine H_1-receptor antagonist.
6. It has a dual action on both serotonin and noradrenaline from the starting dose (30 mg daily).

(b) Indications

1. Treatment of depressive disorders (dosage: 30 mg nocte; this may be increased to 45 mg nocte if further clinical improvement is required or if oversedation occurs; it may be decreased to 15 mg nocte if further sedation is required).

N.B.: *Mirtazapine becomes more sedative as the dosage is decreased due to its antihistaminergic effect predominating over its noradrenergic effect. Conversely, it becomes less sedative as the dosage is increased due to its noradrenergic effect predominating over its antihistaminergic effect.*

(c) Adverse effects

1. Significantly higher incidence of weight gain, cf. placebo – which may be partially due to increased appetite.
2. Significantly higher incidence of drowsiness and excessive sedation, cf. placebo – owing to a strong affinity for histamine H_1-receptors.
3. May lack some serotonin-related side-effects – possibly owing to the blockade of serotonin $5HT_2$-receptors which mediate sexual dysfunction/insomnia/agitation/anxiety and blockade of serotonin $5HT_3$-receptors which mediate nausea/vomiting/headache.
4. Lacks cardiovascular side-effects – owing to a very low affinity for α_1-adrenergic receptors.
5. Lacks anticholinergic side-effects – owing to a very low affinity for muscarinic receptors.
6. Blood pressure monitoring is not required, cf. venlafaxine XL.
7. There is no clinically significant interaction with warfarin, cf. venlafaxineXL.
8. When switching antidepressants, the novel action of mirtazapine reduces the risks of the serotonin syndrome.
9. When switching antidepressants, there is no wash out period usually required with mirtazapine, so patient therapy is not interrupted (except for MAOIs).

VIII. NORADRENALINE REUPTAKE INHIBITORS (NARIs)

Reboxetine (the first NARI) was launched in the UK in 1997.

(a) Mode of action

A highly selective noradrenaline reuptake inhibitor with no significant effect on serotonergic processes.

(b) Indication

Treatment of depression (dosage: 4 mg b.d. in adults; if further clinical improvement is required, this may be increased to 6 mg mane, 4 mg nocte and again if necessary to the maximum dosage of 6 mg b.d. in adults).

(c) Adverse effects

1. Anticholinergic side-effects (e.g. dry mouth, constipation).
2. It is not recommended for use in the elderly.
3. When switching antidepressants, the predominantly noradrenergic action of reboxetine reduces the risk of serotonin syndrome.
4. When switching antidepressants, there is no wash out period usually required with reboxetine, so patient therapy is not interrupted (except for MAOIs).

IX. Pindolol

(a) Indications*

1. Some evidence for treatment of resistant depression as an augmenting agent to SSRIs or dual action SSRIs (by enhancing serotonergic accumulation within the synapse).

*These indications are not currently licensed in the UK.

2. Some evidence for treatment of resistant depression as part of the triple therapy:
   (i) SSRI
   (ii) Buspirone
   (iii) Pindolol

X. THYROXINE

(a) Indications*

1. It may be used to augment antidepressant drug treatment in resistant depression.
2. It may have mood-elevating properties when clinical depression and subclinical hypothyroidism co-exist (the latter being defined as a free thyroxine serum level at the lower end of the normal range).

*These indications are not currently licensed in the UK.

CHAPTER 4

Mood-stabilizing Drugs

I. LITHIUM CARBONATE

(a) Mode of action

The precise mechanism by which lithium produces its therapeutic effect is complex and poorly understood.

Postulated mechanisms of therapeutic effects:

1. Decreased neurotransmitter postsynaptic receptor sensitivity.
2. Stimulates exit of Na^+ from cells where intracellular Na^+ is elevated (as in depression) by stimulating the Na^+/K^+ pump mechanism.
3. Stimulates entry of Na^+ into cells where intracellular Na^+ is reduced (as in mania).
4. Influences Ca^{2+} and Na^+ transfer across cell membranes including the Ca^{2+}-dependent release of neurotransmitter.
5. Inhibits both cyclic AMP and inositol phophate 'second messenger' systems in the membrane – this mechanism mediates the long-term side-effects of nephrogenic diabetes insipidus and hypothyroidism (see below), i.e. lithium blocks ADH-sensitive adenyl cyclase and TSH-sensitive adenyl cyclase, respectively.
6. Interacts with Ca^{2+} and Mg^{2+}, thereby increasing cell membrane permeability.

(b) Indications

1. Treatment of depressive disorders:
   (i) Treatment can be justified in the acute stages of

depressive disorders, when other measures have failed.

(ii) Treatment of resistant depression – i.e. effective in patients who have failed to respond to a cyclic antidepressant drug (mono-, bi-, tri- or tetracyclic antidepressants).

(iii) Enhances the effects of TCAs and MAOIs.

(iv) Enhances the effects of SSRIs – however, lithium should be introduced cautiously because of the risk of the serotonin syndrome developing (owing to enhanced serotonergic activity); this risk appears to be lowest with fluvoxamine.

2. Preventing relapse of depressive disorders:

(i) In unipolar affective disorders:

- Lithium reduces the rate of relapse (but is probably no more effective than continuing TCA treatment).
- After the first episode, treatment should be prolonged for 6 months postclinical recovery.
- After 2 or more episodes – treatment should be prolonged for several (1–3) years post-clinical recovery; lithium is particularly useful in the prophylaxis of recurrent unipolar depression.
- Continuing treatment with lithium reduces the rate of relapse after treatment with ECT.

(ii) In bipolar affective disorders – prolonged administration of lithium (5 years) prevents relapses into depression.

3. Treatment of mania:

Lithium is effective in high doses (1000 mg nocte), but the therapeutic response usually only occurs in the second week of treatment; thus, the response to lithium is slower than the response to antipsychotic drugs.

4. Preventing relapse of mania:
   In bipolar affective disorders, prolonged administration of lithium (5 years) prevents relapses into mania.
5. Treatment of mixed affective states.
6. Prophylaxis of schizoaffective disorders – in combination with an antipsychotic depot injection.
7. Treatment of aggressive or self-mutilating behaviour.

(c) Adverse effects

1. Short-term side-effects:
   (i) Gastrointestinal disturbances (nausea, vomiting, diarrhoea).
   (ii) Fine tremor.
   (iii) Muscle weakness.
   (iv) Polyuria.
   (v) Polydypsia.
2. Long-term side-effects:
   (i) Nephrogenic diabetes insipidus.
   (ii) Hypothyroidism.
   (iii) Cardiotoxicity.
   (iv) Irreversible renal damage (in patients with pre-existing renal pathology).
   (v) Oedema.
   (vi) Weight gain.
   (vii) Tardive dyskinesia and other movement disorders.
3. Toxic effects:
   (i) Increasing gastrointestinal disturbances (anorexia, vomiting, diarrhoea).
   (ii) Increasing CNS disturbances (coarse tremor, drowsiness, ataxia, nystagmus, inco-ordination, slurring of speech, convulsions, coma).
   (iii) The effects of lithium overdosage may be fatal –

hence it is important that the serum lithium level be closely monitored to ensure that it lies within the therapeutic range of 0.4–1.0 mmol/l (the lower end of this range is for maintenance therapy; the higher end of this range is for treatment in the acute stages of illness) on blood samples taken 12 hours after the last dose of lithium; serum lithium levels over 1.5 mmol/l may be fatal.

(iv) Once stabilized on lithium carbonate, the following should be monitored:
- Every 3 months – serum lithium level and serum urea and electrolytes.
- Every 6 months – thyroid functions test.
- Every 12 months – ECG.

N.B.: *Before commencing lithium therapy, baseline investigations should include a serum urea and electrolytes, a thyroid function test and an ECG.*

4. Drug interactions:
   (i) Sodium depletion raises the serum lithium level and may result in lithium toxicity – therefore the concurrent use of diuretics (particularly thiazides) should be avoided.
   (ii) The concurrent use of carbamazepine with lithium may result in neurotoxicity without raising the serum lithium level – hence if carbamazepine is added to lithium, it should be done so with caution – cf. the concurrent use of sodium valproate with lithium which is safe.
   (iii) NSAIDs raise the serum lithium level and may result in lithium toxicity – therefore their concurrent use with lithium should be avoided.
   (iv) ACE inhibitors raise the serum lithium level.

(d) Contraindications:

(i) Pregnancy.
(ii) Breast feeding.
(iii) Renal impairment.

I. CARBAMAZEPINE

Available as a standard formulation requiring three times a day dosing and a modified release formulation (Tegretol Retard) to allow twice daily dosing (up to 800 mg b.d.).

(a) Mode of action

1. Structurally similar to the tricyclic antidepressant imipramine – however, carbamazepine has no effect on monoamine reuptake.
2. Thought to mediate its therapeutic effect by inhibiting kindling phenomena in the limbic system.

(b) Indications

1. Treatment of depressive disorders:
   (i) Treatment of resistant depression, i.e. worth a trial in patients who have failed to respond to a cyclic antidepressant drug and lithium carbonate.
   (ii) Enhances the effects of TCAs and SSRIs.
2. Preventing relapse of depressive disorders:
   (i) It prevents relapses into depression in both recurrent unipolar affective disorders and recurrent bipolar affective disorders.
   (ii) It is the mood stabilizer of choice in patients with both epilepsy and bipolar affective disorder since it also has anticonvulsant properties.
3. Treatment of mania – carbamazepine is effective in

high doses (600 mg b.d.–800 mg b.d.), but the therapeutic response usually only occurs in the second week of treatment; thus, the response to carbamazepine is slower than the response to antipsychotic drugs.

4. Preventing relapse of mania:
   (i) In patients who fail to respond to lithium carbonate – carbamazepine can either be substituted for, or added to, lithium; the two drugs appear to have a synergistic effect when used in combination (but see earlier note on their concurrent use).
   (ii) In patients with the rapid-cycling form of bipolar affective disorder (i.e. four or more affective episodes per year) – carbamazepine is a better prophylactic agent than lithium carbonate.
5. Treatment of all forms of epilepsy – except absence seizures.
6. Treatment of trigeminal neuralgia.
7. Treatment of behavioural disorders secondary to limbic epileptic instability.
8. Treatment of aggressive behaviour (including after head injury).
9. Treatment of acute alcohol withdrawal.

(c) Adverse effects

1. Side-effects:
   (i) Dizziness and drowsiness.
   (ii) Generalized erythematous rash (3%).
   (iii) Visual disturbances (especially double vision).
   (iv) Gastrointestinal disturbances (anorexia, constipation).
   (v) Leucopenia and other blood disorders.
   (vi) Hyponatraemia.
2. Carbamazepine must be initiated at a dosage of 200 mg

b.d. (due to autointroduction, i.e. it often raises the serum level of an active metabolite of carbamazepine) and increased after 1 week to the usual therapeutic dosage of 200 mg mane, 400 mg nocte required for prophylaxis (some patients may require 400 mg b.d.) – carbamazepine is a less toxic drug than lithium carbonate and regular serum level estimation appears to be unnecessary; however, because of the slight risk of leucopenia and other blood disorders, it is important that full blood count is monitored periodically.

3. Carbamazepine is an inducer of the liver enzyme cytochrome P4502D6 – thus it can lower plasma haloperidol levels by half.
4. Carbamazepine also decreases the plasma concentration of:
   (i) Oral contraceptives.
   (ii) Warfarin.
5. The plasma concentration of carbamazepine is increased by:
   (i) Erythromycin.
   (ii) Cimetidine.
   (iii) Calcium-channel blockers.
   (iv) Isoniazid.
6. The plasma concentration of carbamazepine is reduced by:
   Phenytoin.

N.B.: *The maximum dosage of carbamazepine is 800 mg b.d. (prescribed as Tegratol Retard).*

II. SODIUM VALPROATE/ VALPROATE SEMISODIUM

Sodium valproate is available as a standard formulation requiring three times a day dosing and a modified release formulation (Epilim Chrono) to allow twice daily dosing (up to 1200 mg b.d.).

N.B.: *Valproate semisodium (comprising of equimolar amounts of Sodium Valproate and Valproic Acid) is currently licensed in the UK and USA for bipolar affective disorder. Sodium valproate has also been used, but it is unlicensed for this indication. In terms of cost, valproate semisodium is approximately five times more expensive than Sodium Valproate (prescribed as Epilim Chrono) for equivalent dosages.*

(a) Mode of action

1. Sodium valproate is thought to mediate its therapeutic effect through indirect effects on GABA-ergic systems (i.e. it may slow GABA breakdown by inhibiting succinic semialdehyde dehydrogenase), implicating a possible underlying biochemical disturbance of GABA deficiency in some affective disorders.
2. Valproate semisodium is thought to permeate the blood brain barrier more easily, cf. sodium valproate – this, in turn, results in a higher concentration of valproate in the brain with valproate semisodium, cf. an equivalent dose of sodium valproate.

(b) Indications

1. Treatment of depressive disorders:
   (i) Treatment of resistant depression, i.e. worth a trial

in patients who have failed to respond to a cyclic antidepressant drug, lithium carbonate and carbamazepine.

(ii) Enhances the effects of TCAs and SSRIs.

2. Preventing relapse of depressive disorders – they prevent relapses into depression in bipolar affective disorders.
3. Treatment of mania – sodium valproate is effective in high doses (600 mg b.d. – 1200 mg b.d.), but the therapeutic response usually only occurs in the second week of treatment; thus, the response to sodium valproate is slower than the response to antipsychotic drugs.

N.B.: *With valproate semisodium, the therapeutic response is claimed to occur in the first week of treatment, cf. sodium valproate [the dosing for valproate semisodium is 750* mg *daily in divided doses (day one), then 500* mg *b.d. to 1000* mg *b.d. or 20* mg*/kg/day from day two onwards].*

4. Preventing relapse of mania:
   (i) Effective as a mood stabilizer in some manic patients who fail to respond to lithium carbonate and carbamazepine.
   (ii) In the case of lithium carbonate, sodium valproate can be safely added to it and has been shown to enhance the effectiveness of lithium as a mood stabilizer.
   (iii) May also be used as a first line treatment – on both clinical and litigation grounds, valproate semisodium should be preferred to sodium valproate.
5. Treatment of all forms of epilepsy.

N.B.: *It is better to prescribe valproate semisodium as the brand depakote, to avoid confusion with sodium valproate.*

(c) Adverse effects

1. Side-effects:
   (i) Recent concern over severe hepatic and pancreatic toxicity.
   (ii) Haematological disturbance (thrombocyto-penia, inhibition of platelet aggregation).
   (iii) Drowsiness, weight gain and hair loss.
2. Sodium valproate is initiated at a dosage of 200 mg b.d. and increased after 1 week to 400 mg b.d. and again after another week to 600 mg b.d., the usual therapeutic dosage required for prophylaxis (some patients may require 800 mg b.d.) – sodium valproate is a less toxic drug than lithium and regular serum level estimation appears to be unnecessary; however, because of the slight risk of severe hepatic toxicity, severe pancreatic toxicity and haematological disturbance of platelet function, it is important that liver function tests, serum amylase level and full blood count are monitored periodically.

N.B.: *The maximum dosage of sodium valproate is 1200 mg b.d. (prescribed as Epilim Chrono).*

NOTES

NOTES